Erbs Palsy and Me

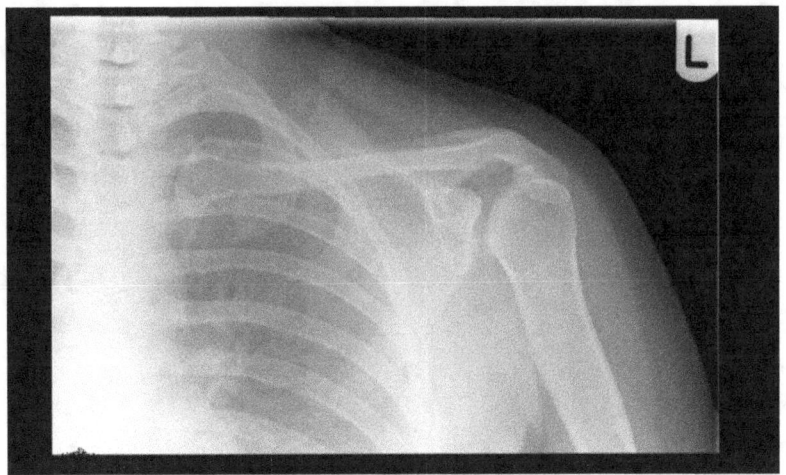

Real Life Honest Comedic View of what it's like to
live with an Erbs Palsy Birth Injury

Ms. F.U ARM

Warning Contains Honest Language

.

CHAPTERS

7. Working

8. Having Children

9. Prognoses

1. Who am I?

Who am I?

I'm 39 years old born in South Wales in the UK

I'm a valleys girl by heart. I sustained a serious life changing birth injury in August 1979 in a Welsh City Hospital not naming any names here.

My mother went through hours of agony giving birth to me with doctors hovering over her pushing on her belly with another pulling on my neck to get me out.

I was a 9lb baby big but not unusually big they knew i was big and my mother was having problems giving birth to me as I was stuck, she should have been rushed in for a caesarian section, I haven't spoken about it much with my mother as it was very traumatic for her so I'm only telling you what I know. The moment I was worn I was whisked off straight away with my arm all flopping everywhere, my poor mother didn't have a clue what was going on she thought I was dead.

My mother to this day still hasn't a clue exactly what is or was wrong with me. When I was diagnosed with Erbs palsy and well enough to go home my parents were advised by the doctors in the hospital to tie my arm to the side of the cot so that my arm

would heal and set properly, very medieval.
Little did they know the terrible effects it would cause me later on in life.

Back in 1979 there was no help and no proper explanation as to what was wrong with me , I never had any physiotherapy at all , I never crawled as a baby as I could only bum shuffle everywhere which I think has contributed to my back problems later in life .

I do remember as a child going back and forth the hospital just for them to check my progress, but never any treatment offered or advised.

I'd sit there as a child while this old cold handed doctor with a hammer used to come and hit me on the arms and the legs, that old bastard did some mental damage I think. I remember the one year on my checkup I was asked to have a photo taken of me in a standing position so they could see the progress I had been making.

The only thing was they wanted me a little girl to take her vest off , no way I screamed the place down , even at that age I understood that it was wrong of some guy to take my top off and ask me to stand there half naked whilst he takes photos of me. I played holy hell my mother had to make another appointment when my father was off work to take me. My Dad did take me and I got to keep my vest on. I was only around 6 when this happened after this time I cannot remember going to see anyone else up until the age of 21 when I had my first x ray of my shoulder.

2. What is Erbs Palsy?

So what is Erbs Palsy, there are many different variations of the Bracial plexus injury from birth and this is what I've learnt myself.

Erbs palsy is also known as obstetric brachial plexus palsy as a result of an injury at birth known as shoulder dystocia as a result of the baby's shoulders being stuck against the mother's pelvic bone in the uterus.
The baby's head is pulled at the neck at different angles to release the baby from the pelvis thus resulting in the stretching and tearing of the nerves. I can imagine the doctors were pulling me left and right like a bloody cork in a bottle.

The network of nerves that lay in the neck known as the bracial plexus these are roots that come out of the spinal cord and fuses to the collarbone. The nerves are very import and control the muscle movement in the arm to the shoulder down to the elbow then wrist and hand.

The variations are given grades from 1 to 4 in disability and recovery prognosis.
I'm what's known as a grade 4, I have permanent irreversible damage which left untreated as mine has develops into other disabilities years down the line.

Diagram Spinal Colum Nerve Roots

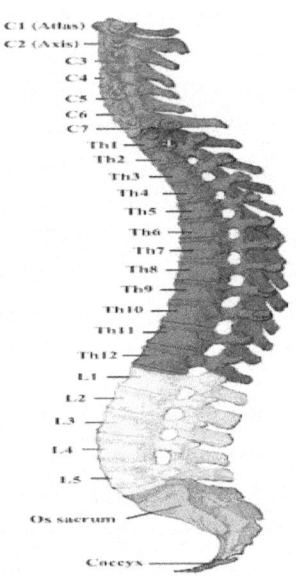

In the UK the primary classification system is called the Narakas classification system which was developed by A.O. Narakas in 1986

The Narakas classification system

Group 1: Group 1 represents injury to the C5 and C6 nerve roots resulting in:

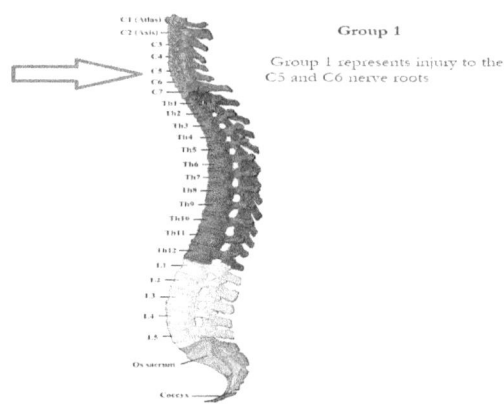

- Difficulty lifting the affected arm above the head (restricted shoulder abduction)
- Difficulty rotating the shoulder away from the body (restricted external rotation)
- Difficulty bending the elbow (restricted elbow flexion)
- Difficulty twisting the forearm so that the palm of the hand is facing forward (restricted forearm supination).

As a result, a person with brachial plexus injury may present with the affected arm hanging down by their side, straightened and rotated towards the body, and with the palm of the hand facing backwards in pronation.

90% of people with a group 1 injury will return to having normal function.

Group 2: Group 2 represents injury to the C5, C6 and C7 nerve roots. In addition to the difficulties experienced above, people in group 2 also have difficulty in bending the wrist back (wrist extension).

75% of people with a group 2 injury will return to having normal function.

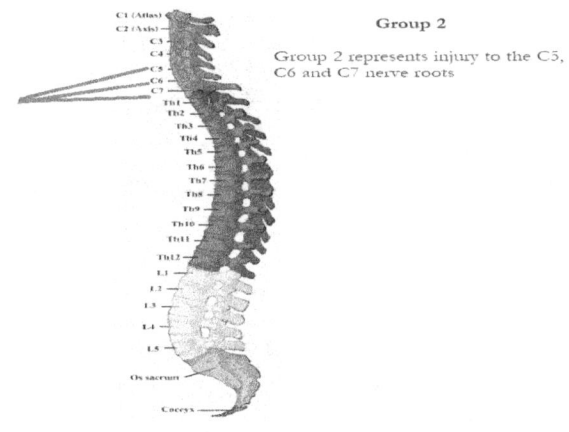

Group 2

Group 2 represents injury to the C5, C6 and C7 nerve roots

Group 3: Group 3 represents injury to the C5, C6, C7 and C8 nerve roots. People in this group experience complete arm paralysis.

Less than 50% recover some satisfactory function.

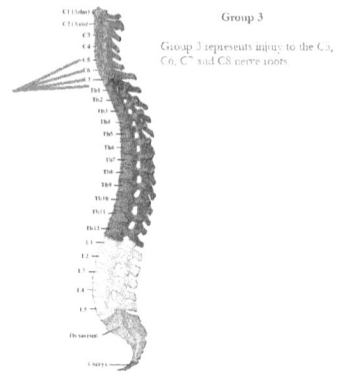

Group 4: Group 4 represents injury to the C5, C6, C7, C8 and T1 nerve roots. In addition to arm paralysis, people in group 4 experience Horner's syndrome. Horner's syndrome describes damage to a bundle of nerves that are responsible for controlling some of the muscles of the eye. As a result, people with Horner's syndrome have a constricted pupil and droopy eyelid.

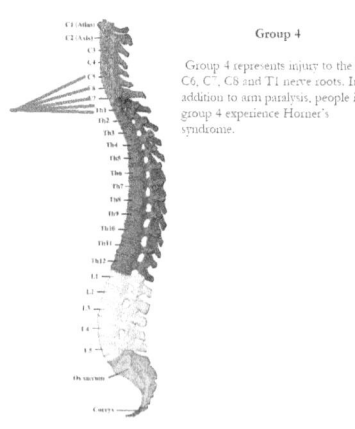

I fall into the Group 4 as I have damage to the T1 and T2 nerve roots and droopy eye as displayed in Horners syndrome.

3. My Erbs Palsy

If I'm truly honest with you this is the beginning of my search to find out what exactly is wrong with me.

Erbs palsy is not just a birth injury that you just get over; there are long lasting disabilities that never get spoken about.

Do you know how hard it is to find any information on Erbs palsy in adults and the long lasting issues and consequences of birth injuries through medical negligence?

I was diagnosed with Erbs palsy at birth, but the symptoms that I have show's I have Klumpskes palsy and Horners syndrome as well, try telling people and they think you're dying from some unknown disease.

My left has very limited movement global wasting of the left shoulder and arm musculature. Brachial radials reflexes are absent and no external rotation. My shoulder is hypo plastic (under grown) with degenerate damage.

I cannot lift my arm above my chest or rotate my wrist, I tend to hold my arm to my chest as it protrudes a little at the elbow and I tend to bang into things with it. I don't have the recognized claw hand as with Klumpskes palsy but I do have damage to the T1 and T2 nerves.

I have a slight droop to me left eye and issues with weak muscles in my eyes which I wear glasses for but I look trendy in them lol.

I have hypertrophy (over growth) of the ligamentum flavum posteriorly as the L4/5 and L5/S1 causing mild reduction on canal diameter posteriorly. Incidentally there is a high signal focus on T2 axial's in the right hand side of S1 which on sagittal images appears to be of similar signal on T1 and T2 . This was confirmed as haemangioma try saying that mouthful to someone.

The following are my own personal X ray's and

MRI

4. X Rays and MRI scans

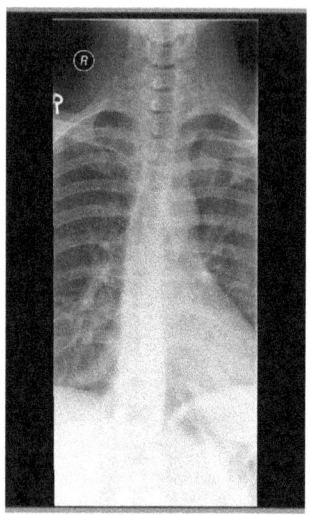

X Rays taken in 2015 report I have a slight lumber scoliosis concave to the right

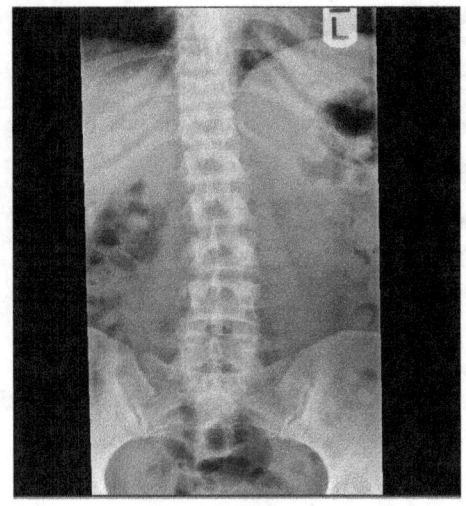

MRI taken in 2015

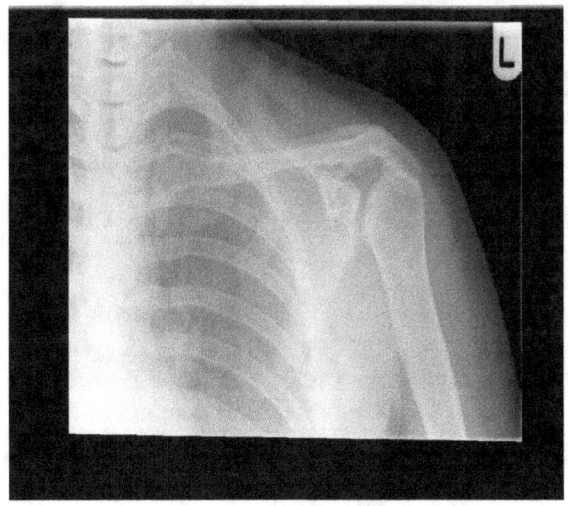

Left Shoulder x ray Taken in 2007

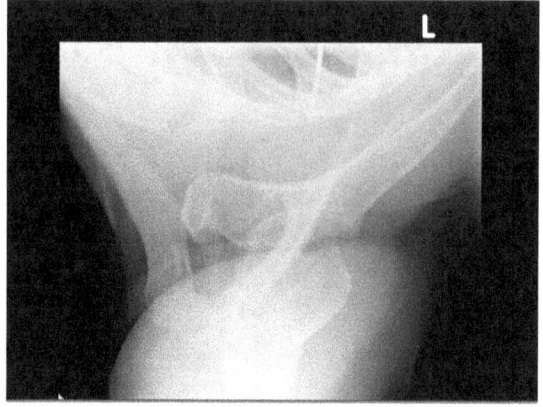

Left Shoulder x ray Taken 2007

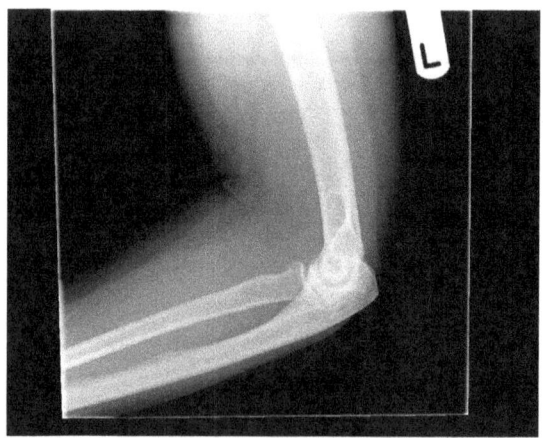

Left Elbow x ray – I've been told my elbow is normal

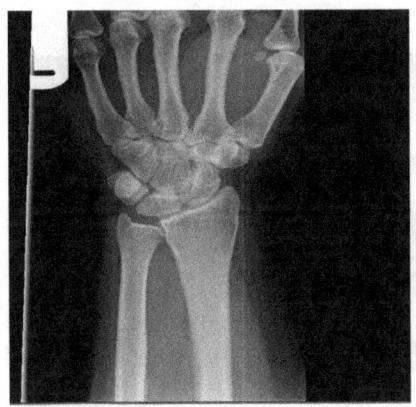

Left wrist x ray 2007 I've been told this is a
normal x Ray and my wrist is fine, however I
cannot rotate my wrist

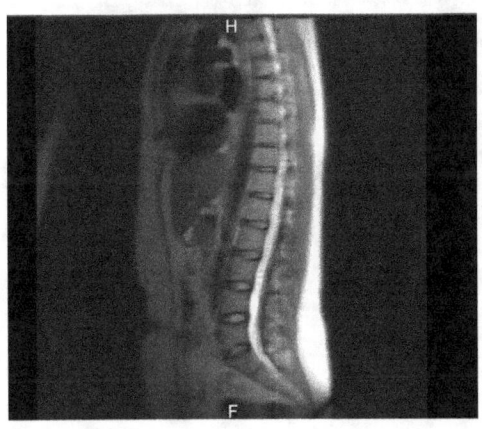

MRI of my spine 2015

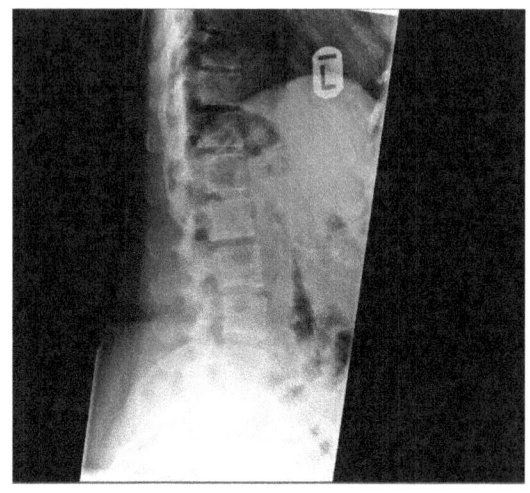

x ray of my Lower Lumber 2007

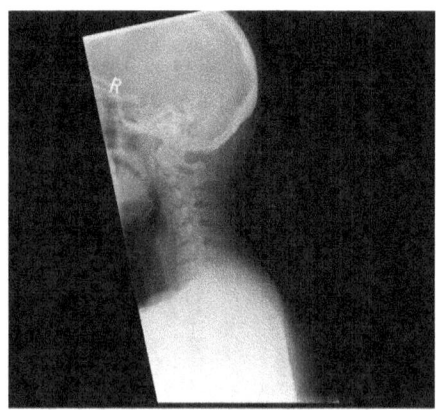

Head and Neck x ray Taken 2007

5. Growing up

It wasn't easy growing up with Erbs palsy, you're not able to do the things that normal abled children do. Simple things like juggle a ball or do a hand stand or even put your coat on properly without looking like a tit like you have some Michael Jackson move going on out of thriller.

The number of funny stares I've had for just putting my coat on you wouldn't believe.

If you have a child with Erbs palsy just a bit of advice don't pick them up under the arms it really hurts , that's one thing I hated as a child being picked up , the pain is unbearable.

Early school life was a nightmare I don't remember much about infants and juniors I hated school early years. I was always taking time off school.

I remember when I first started junior school after we had moved in from over the other valley so I had no choice in the matter this was my new school. It was just after the miner's strike I remember going for the disgusting dinners in the school holidays with your yellow meal tickets.

My dad had left the pit and got himself a new job we had a new house in the neighboring valley I could see my old house from our back garden. It was great where I lived we were in a new build, It was the first set of semi on the plot, I remember the cold concrete floors and having to share a room with my brother until the house had been decorated.

New job new house new life, but for me it was new house new job more holidays same life different school.

I hated school even as a baby in nursery school I remember hanging off my mother's neck when she dropped me off for nursery with Mrs. Davis with the massive bee hive hair door. I was terrified of her hair doo I used to think she has real bees living in her hair, she was a big build old fashioned red headed welsh woman , very scary and very loud.

I painfully remember my first day at Junior school, yes I will name and shame you our head mistress was Miss Jones, I was sat with the other children in the assembly hall after my mother had just brought me to school, Miss Jones asked me to stand up in assembly so she could introduce me to the school children on my first day.

Ofmg if she could ever do anything worse I felt like a right tit , she only went and told everyone I had the DISEASE called Erbs palsy it was most probably downfall of my early school years.

From that day on everyone thought that I had a disease that they would catch the dodgy arm disease, lol and to top it off I was a red head so that with a dodgy arm in school kids used to run from me thinking they would catch it.

Yeah thanks Miss Jones I hate you!

I hardly went to school I used to walk myself down the lane to school get half way then turn around and come back home, it even got to the extent that I used to put my head on the radiator to say that I had a temperature so that I didn't have to go to school.

I was and am still very aware of how my arm looks I hate having my photo taken still to this day I will look at it and the first thing my eyes turn to is how dodgy my arm looks .

At home though I had a great childhood I lived on the side of the mountain so had the freedom to just go for a wander over the mountain. My mother used to go nuts because she could never find me, I was always off on my travels normally with my sheepdog and Siamese cat in tow.

I was very selective of my friends as a young girl and because of my disability it allowed me to grow up that little bit tougher.

If truth be told I think the crap i had growing up from other kids has mentally and emotionally scared me for life.

I was always happy when I was around adults, there was a man that lived up the lane his name was Dai he used to ride motorbikes, I spent most of my time over the summer in the garage with him stripping his big Yamaha super bike or flying his petrol model helicopter. The noise of the helicopter used to drive my mother nuts but I didn't care I thought it was awesome.

I spent allot of time in the summers with my grandparents whilst my parents were in work where I learnt practical skills in life. My grandfather was a champion gardener with his local village allotment club or what is known as clickyville allot of clicky old men who like to chat about each other's marrows.

I used to love helping him in the garden digging shit planting flowers and getting high on paraffin fumes in his green house in the winter, and laughing at his three legged giant carrots and parsnips.

I used to love it in spring when all the daffodils were in full bloom my grandfather used to have the as edging around his lawn, when they were at the end of their bloom me and my brother used to run and do karate kicks at them trying to hit the heads off as we jumped over them, I think that may have been down to playing too much street fighter thinking back on it.

He taught me all my gardening skills, he even taught me to knit. So you could say that my grandfather set me up for later in life as now I'm self-employed and I grow plants , I make my own wooden jewellery from the wood grown in my own garden and knit clothes and fashion accessories to sell online . So thanks Dad (that's what I call him).

I did learn to play the guitar which I can still play a little now but due to the fast cord change I found it impossible to move my arm fast enough up the neck of the guitar.

My father taught me the basics I also had paid for lessons but had to stop as it was too painful and could have been doing more damage to my arm. Luckily though I have two sons who are self-taught so I have the pleasure of being proud mum listening to them play.

I do however play piano , I started playing 2 years ago as a physio for my arm, it's still slow but hey I can now play piano and I'm not bad if truth be told , as long as I don't have to play anything fast lol I'm fucked then ha ha.

I hated sports apart from swimming , I never participated in any sports in infants or junior school , I was aware that my arm used to stick out when I was running so instead of having the piss taken I just never did it. I did used to get allot of joint pain when I was a child in my knees and my back so I had the excuse not to do it.

I guess if I had a better introduction in school and less of the piss take I would have been participating in school sports.

Outside of school though I was always very sporty id always run everywhere , I was never inside I was always out walking or riding my bike or climbing trees making camps.

The best thing as a child I did which did improve the range off movement in my arms was swimming, my mother sent me to swimming lessons over the school summer holidays when I was around 9.

I think, I loved it was very little strain on my arm and built up the muscle strength in my arm and shoulder. I was swimming the mile and doing my life saving badges within a few weeks which was handy as I was determined to learn to swim before we went on our holidays to Majorca thanks to Dads new job.

My comprehensive school was connected to the local swimming pool and sports center so I took up swimming for the school swimming team in fact I was captain, the bull they used to call me.

Believe it or not when in water I had the ability to do back stroke the water gave me the force I needed to push with my arm to allow me to raise my arm above my head , out of the water though you got no chance. I captain of the school swimming team, I think my Nan still has the photos of my stood as a skinny teenager in my swimming costume stood by the poolside for the local rag newspaper.

I was always a bit of a tom boy never a girly girl I have an older brother who I spent a lot of time with growing up playing with cars and hanging around with the same mates mostly boys, as a girl hanging around with boys that was just another thing I had stick for but to be honest I didn't give a shit I was enjoying life.

I loved comprehensive school I think it allowed me to be myself more, I still hated sports though. I had little option in comp we had to participate, let's put it this way I got into writing myself notes for the teacher from my mother excusing me from games. I was always made an example of when we had someone come to the school and visit our games lesson as if they were accommodating my needs for my disability, they wasn't really.

I had good male and female friends in comprehensive schools had less slack plus I was finding my own voice in school. I was changing and becoming a crazy hormonal teenager. I think I just came to a point in my life where you just crack you don't take any more crap from the name calling.

I had my first fight at the age of 13 id had enough this girl was taking the mic of my arm so I just flipped walked up to her grabbed her head by her hair and smashed her in the face with me knee .

Lol as you can imagine I never got hassled again. I do think it's important that a child sticks up for themselves there's only a certain amount of crap a child can take , I think that if I didn't crack then I wouldn't be the care free outspoken person that I am now .

I did everything that a normal teenager did in those days omg I'm only 39.

I was a very strong and determined teenager at the age of 15 I was applying for jobs , I couldn't wait to get myself a job and my own independence, I wrote so many letters asking if there was any vacancies.

Because I was born in August I was only 15 when I finished my exams, I didn't want to hang around in life I wanted a job I wanted to drive. I started college two weeks after I finished school.

Mechanical engineering through the summer school operating big industrial lathe machines and doing bench work making tools it was awesome I loved it.

I did have issues with my arm lifting the big heavy chucks onto the lathes but I didn't care if it hurt I was determined that I wouldn't have any help from anyone.

I was very proud of myself because I was good at it and passed my courses with distinction. Some of the boys hated it that I had better grades than them but I will admit the most of the class and tutors were great. Mr. Dartch was my engineering tutor he was great, he used to call me Penelope pit stop.

After mechanical engineering I went on and did welding and electrical engineering which I didn't complete because one of the companies I had written a letter to had offered me an interview. It was in an electrical wholesaler, me wanting to drive I needed the job for my new car so I grabbed the opportunity and loved it.

Learning to drive was an experience, my dad bought me an X Reg Red Austin metro it was great my own first car. I was only 16 at the time so I wasn't allowed to drive it until the day I hit 17. But I nagged my dad to teach me.

We used to keep the metro locked up in the garage at the bottom of the late it wasn't big enough to swing a cat around in. I used to drive out of the garage and up the lane; first to second gear was a breeze. I then used to reverse all the way back down the lane back into the garage; I did this for around 3 months or so.

On my 17th birthday my dad woke me up at 5am to go out early morning before he went to work so I could drive first thing on my 17th birthday. I had 7 2 hour lessons over a two week period and then went for my test at the end of the month.

When I applied of my driving license I didn't apply for the disabled driving license as I didn't classify myself as disabled , yes I was in pain yes I couldn't do the things that others could do but that's one thing I never did classify myself as .

So when I finished my first driving test to be told by the instructor that I had issues with my hand positioning on the steering wheel and that I had failed I was heartbroken as it went all so well I thought I did great. So after going home and telling my parents they instantly booked me up for another test. I had to wait another month for the test as being in September it's a buys time of the year everyone coming of age wanting to do their test like me.

So when I got to the testing station and realized I had the same test instructor my heart sank, he had recognized me from last month so I explained what was wrong with me and he said that I should have told him. I was scared they would put me in for a different test for my disability. Anyways he passed me and actually apologized that he hasn't passed me the first time.

I drove a manual car for years I did suffer I would be out driving and my arm would lock up so I would have to wait for the pain and muscle contraction to ease before I drove again. It was painful driving , I drive an automatic now which is allot easier than a manual but after around 10 -15 miles of driving my arm hurts , so I don't tend to travel very far . Any long distance driving I always have to have someone with me just in case.

6. Daily life

As I've grown older my condition has become worse, years of untreated issues not knowing exactly what was wrong with me, all I knew is what I could do and what I couldn't do.

What I can and can't do

I can't do simple things like cut a steak or peel a potato. I cannot rotate my left wrist to hold say an apple to peal it.

I never go out for meals as I cannot cut my meat and being a meat eater it's not a nice feeling having your other half having to cut up your meat like a baby. If I were to try and do it would even make myself look even more stupid like a cavewoman in a steak house. So I hate going out for meals.

I can't lift any pan to drain it off or lift something heavy out of the oven as I don't have the strength in my arm to do it as it's too painful. I find when my left arm is totally out of commission due to using it then I find I over compensate which causes pain in my right wrist so I can't win either way.

I can't dry my hair with a hair dryer or style my hair properly, its either down or up that's it, now up more often or not as my dog tries to eat my hair, yes it's not nice having a 30lb Cane Corso puppy hanging off your hair she's only 4 months old wish me luck lol.

I have to force my arm above my head sitting on my bum with my arm resting on my knee, it hurts too much it forces my shoulder out of its joint I'm sure, it grinds when I do it its horrible. Over the years my shoulder has gotten worse from the shoulder degradation of use over the years.

so I tend to not dry my hair anymore I just leave it dry on its own naturally which takes a few hours as its down past my bum. I tell my youngest son that I'm a witch and that's why I have long ha ha.

I can't wear a bra so I go el natural, I have never been able to find a bra that fits me properly they always pull down on my shoulder giving me a bad neck and a bad back, I only wear a bra when I go out my boppers are not the smallest so it saves on the stares and awkward glances when my boobs are flopping around in Asda lol.

Because of the position I have kept my arm in over the years close into my chest and the dip in my shoulder I suffer allot of back pain , I constantly feel as if I'm twisted especially when I'm sat down, I have been through years of pain with un comfy chairs and mattresses.

When sitting down to watch Tv I have to put my legs up to get comfy my back arches forward and I have to constantly change my seating position because I have pain in my coccyx , my bum goes numb and my feet and my legs go dead.

 I spend most of the time on the floor sat with my legs crossed but constantly changing my seating position

 I east my food on the floor as it's easier for me to eat sat in this position than having to reach up to the table.

I can't lay on my front as this causes radiating shooting pains from the back off my neck shooting up into my skull.

Because of the curvature of my spine I find it hard to get comfy in bed at night I am constant shifting my position too long on my back and it feels like my back is coming through my chest, I can't sleep on my left hand side as its painful putting pressure on my arm, Its painful sleeping on my side because I have issues with my hips.

I cannot touch my arm or put pressure on certain parts of my body even hovering a hand or anything over my arm or shoulder sets of the shooting nerve pain that is unbearable. My skin feels like I've been bruised when touched.

I get days where I just don't get dressed because it's too painful lifting my arm or problems lifting my legs to put on clothes when my hips or knees play up , yes I have arthritis of the hips and knees also.

Some days I just mosh around in my nightie because I just can't be bothered with the pain. I think there is a certain point in your life where there are no days free of pain it's always something or another.

I've tried many different prescribed drugs over the years in dealing with my pain. I don't like being monged out on tramadol and fed up off gut problems with taken ibuprofen for many years I decided to try a different approach.

I have never found a pain killer comparable to that of cannabis; it's the best pain killer I have found that deals with the constant dull ache and stabbing nerve pain.

I went to my doctor and asked if I could be

prescribed Sativex and all I got was what's that I've never heard of it. The doctor doesn't seem to care, your sat there explaining what's wrong with you all whilst the doctor is looking at a computer screen, I gave up on my doctor years ago, I have issues wrong with me that I haven't even spoken to the doctor about because I feel what's the point they make you feel like a hypochondriac when I have genuine issues.

For example back a few years ago I was going back and fore the doctors with issues of IBS heart palpitations and pains in my stomach and bloating etc my stomach was really bloated at the time I looked pregnant, doctor felt my stomach and said it was fat lol , so my partner rushed me to hospital, turns out it was my pancreas now I have scarring inside from the damage that was done because i was left untreated.

I've been telling my doctor for years I can't feel my legs my feet go blue , but nothing it was only because I had complained about my back that I was sent for the x rays and MRI that I found out exactly why my legs back and feet go dead, this should have been dealt with years ago.

So no i don't have any confidence in the doctors or medical industry what so ever because as far as I'm concerned I have been let down from the moment my mother went into hospital to give birth to me. I can't do anything about this now legally because I'm too old to make a claim even though everything I know I had to find out myself, it's like as if I have been held back with my condition and my plea's to find out what is exactly wrong with me has been ignored.

The damage is done now and I just have to live with it. So if I sound angry and resentful it's because I am and I quite entitled to be.

I have been self-medicating with cannabis now for over 15 years and I will never go back to prescribed medication for my Erbs pain again.
I smoke it but for those who don't smoke it can eat it , yes it is illegal but I don't care , ive done my research and experienced the benefits so if someone wants to criticize me for alleviate my pain with a natural herb then they need to do more research. Its not legal here but it's getting there that one day everyone will be able to treat their conditions with legal cannabis.

If I didn't self-medicate with cannabis I wouldn't be able to cope with the little work I do now, I am self-employed everything I earn with the pain of using my own hands of which I am proud of as I don't claim any benefits even though I am entitled to them I would rather have the satisfaction that I did it on my own.

As I've grown older the pain has become worse. I find myself walking less going out driving less its hard work I get worn out real easy.

Sitting down is uncomfortable standing up is uncomfortable it's as if I was cursed to keep moving to stay comfy which makes things worse.

The simple thing of standing at the mirror in the bathroom putting on your lippy leaning forward hurts my lower back my neck and my legs go dead and blue.

I've been told that what damage is done has been done and cannot be fixed and will only get worse , I'm 39 years old and feel as if I'm in my 60's and the thought that it's only going to get worse I think is kind of terrifying. Most of all having to ask my other half to do things for me because I can't I feel useless.

7. Working

I do work I'm self-employed , I worked for other people for many years and found that companies don't like or appreciate you taking time off work because your arm is locked up or your having problems with your back and you can't move without shooting pains running down your leg from your but with every step or movement you take.

I gave up counting on anyone else so I started my own little business I took the skills that my grandfather taught me and started growing plants to sell online , I had massive help from my kids and my other half who without them I wouldn't be able to run a profitable online business. I also make handmade jewellery and knit socks and headwear on my drill powered loom machine so I don't even have to make the effort to knit now thanks to my other half it's all done by machine. It is painful I only work around 1 to 2 hours a day as that's all I can manage so I have my fingers in many pies I don't make that much but I make enough to pay the bills. It's a struggle sometimes but that's life.

8. Having children

I have 4 kids 3 boys and girl who's a right tom boy. On my first son I had terrible trouble with the birth due to me having high blood pressure, I had an epidural and was getting ready for a caesarean section but lucky I didn't need one.

It was scary having my first child as there was a possibility of happening what happened to me, it was the same hospital same ward and under the same doctor funny enough. I spent a lot of my time during the birth of my oldest son reading my old medical records looking at my old hand written notes with my left hand as a child, my midwife was amazed my life story played out before her as I was having my first child having complications of my own on the same ward in the same hospital under the same doctor.

It was uncanny, funny enough I never did get to see my doctor, I wonder why.

I've now stopped at 4 children and I can honestly say it's been painful having to deal with the inability to breast feed because I could never position my arm to sort the baby, even lifting the baby's legs to change a nappy was painful but you struggle on and just get on with the job that needs to be done and deal with the pain later.

I've never been able to have the kids cuddle up under my arm I've never been able to pick them up or play with them without being in pain , but I wouldn't change things for the world. My oldest has now just turned 20 and my youngest is 10 so I haven't done badly over the years in managing thanks to the help of my other half who has been an amazing dad to all our children.

9. Prognoses

My condition will only become worse as the years pass by and I have accepted that, all I can do is learn to adapt to my disabilities. I've told my other half the day I can't wipe my own arse put me out of it ha ha.

I hope I have helped those who have children with Erbs palsy what their long term prognosis could be. It would have been nice to have been table to talk to someone about my condition to understand exactly what was wrong with me, and understanding why my arse is hurting so much sat down typing this on my little laptop believe me my arse is numb and I can't feel my back from my neck down, so I hope I have helped others who are going through the same issues as me.

I do blame the hospital for my condition and the lack of help and education , the first time I had access to the internet at the age of 16 my first web search was " what is erbs palsy " , I was the one that was educating my parents on my disabilities when it should have been the other way around. I had no help what so ever, and still don't I keep getting referred to doctors and orthopedic surgeons who have no experience in my condition at all , its like been passed from pillar to post , even then they never properly explain what's wrong with you. The last orthopedic specialist I seen about my condition wrote on the report that I had no issues sleeping at night which was the complete opposite of what I had told him, he also stated that there is no numbness when I specifically told him I had issues, he also failed to tell me I had two Spinal hemangiomas one on my neck and one on my lower. I only found this information out by obtaining my medical records which most of them are still missing.

I wouldn't be the person I am today if I didn't have my condition. I feel that my disabilities could have been prevented with early treatment but we are talking about the late 70's early 80's so we weren't as much in the know about this as we are now.

Well I've had enough now so thanks for taking the time to read my little story , I never went to school much so my grammar is pretty rubbish but I don't give a toss lol .

ACKNOWLEDGMENTS

The World Wide Web for helping me understand what exactly what Erbs Palsy is without you I wouldn't know any different?

And most of all my partner he who is always there for me, if it wasn't for him I wouldn't be writing this now.

DEDICATION

To all the Erbs Palsy sufferers who has been asking questions all their lives but still waiting for the answers

Erbs Palsy and Me

Erbs Palsy and Me

Erbs Palsy and Me

ABOUT THE AUTHOR

An honest representation of living with Erbs Palsy
the highs and the lows of living with a life changing
birth injury

Born in South Wales UK 1979 Ms F.U Arm